FERTILE PATH

NAVIGATING INFERTILITY WITH UNDERSTANDING AND HOPE

DR. WHITNEY DAVID

ISBN: 9798879312737

DEDICATION

This book is dedicated to everyone who has struggled with infertility. To every man and woman who has experienced the agony of erratic menstrual cycles, the fragility of medical examinations, and the challenges of managing pharmaceutical regimens: To the brave souls who have battled to become fearless, flexible, and reliable parents.

I hope that you find comfort, understanding, and a sense of belonging on these pages. I hope they remind you of the fact you are not alone on this journey. May they assist you in discovering your own prosperous path, led by empathy and comprehension.

I hope you find solace, understanding, and a feeling of community inside these pages. I hope they serve as a reminder of the fact you cannot do it alone. May they guide you to your own prosperous journey with care and optimism.

CONTENTS

ACKNOWLEDGMENTS

In making "Fertile path," I am filled with gratitude for the remarkable individuals who walked alongside me. I stand on the shoulders of quite a large number. My family's relentless help, friends and fellow warriors fighting the same expectation, and my great team insight formed this excursion. May these pages provide readers seeking solace with understanding, comfort and hope.

ASKING FOR ASSISTANCE ON THE FERTILE PATH

Introduction

The path to infertility is difficult and sometimes feels vague and meandering. The road to motherhood may be physically and emotionally draining for individuals who aspire to be parents. However, despite the difficulties, hope endures a light that shines through the deepest shadows. We travel through the challenges of infertility in Fertile Paths. We understand that asking for assistance is a brave step towards comprehension and resolution, rather than a sign of weakness. Let's examine the value of prompt action, the effectiveness of medical advice, and the possibility of optimism.

The Quiet Battle

Couples may struggle with unsaid anxieties and question why they are unable to conceive. However, we don't have to be alone and quiet. We create opportunities by admitting we struggle and getting help from professionals. The Function of Health Care Practitioners Our allies become medical professionals, reproductive experts, and nurses. They hear our tales, solve the enigmas around our bodies, and point us in the direction of solutions. Their proficiency converts doubt into understanding, and understanding enables us to make well-informed choices.

Early Intervention: A Gift Time is both a friend and an enemy. Early intervention gives people hope. It enables us to locate the root issues, deal with them right away, and consider our alternatives for therapy. Early assistance helps us take back control of our story. A Mutual Understanding Community We come together as a group in this book a circle of compassionate hearts. We encourage one another, exchange tales, and bust myths. We walk the maze of infertility together, knowing that understanding and compassion will guide us. In summary as you peruse these pages, dear reader, keep in mind that you are not alone. Seek assistance, hold on to hope, and bravely stroll the fruitful roads. This is where comprehension and possibilities converge to begin our adventure. With understanding and hope, may your path bring you the joy you want and your heart find comfort.

CAUSES, RISK FACTORS AND DIAGNOSIS OF INFERTILITY

Women's infertility causes

Disorders of Ovulation: Unbalanced hormones might cause irregular ovulation. Conditions like polycystic ovarian syndrome (PCOS) or abnormal hormone levels can prevent the ovaries from releasing mature eggs. Common symptoms include irregular menstrual periods, anovulation, or insufficient ovulation.

Abnormalities of the Uterus or Cervix: Structural issues pertaining to the uterus or cervix can impact fertility. Examples include scarring that prevents a fertilized egg from implanting, polyps, or uterine fibroids.

Endometriosis: Endometriosis is caused by tissue that resembles the lining of the uterus growing outside of it. It may have an impact on fertility by causing adhesions, discomfort, and inflammation.

Obesity: Being overweight might interfere with ovulation and upset the hormonal balance. Reproductive health requires maintaining a healthy weight.

Men Infertility Causes

Low motility of sperm count:
The term "sperm count" describes the quantity of sperm in a sample of semen. A low sperm count makes fertilization less likely to be effective. Sperm motility, or the ability to swim, is a factor in how well they can enter and pierce the egg.

Undescended Testicles: The generation of sperm may be impacted if testicles do not descend correctly during foetal development. It could be necessary to have surgery to fix it.

Genetic Deviations and Hormone Problems:
Hormone dysregulation or genetic abnormalities may affect the quantity and quality of sperm.
Thyroid issues and diabetes are examples of conditions that might be involved.

Diseases and Inflammation: Sexually transmitted infections such as chlamydia and gonorrhea can cause damage to sperm. Inflammation of the reproductive tract may impair fertility.

Factors at Risk for Infertility The several risk factors that might raise the chance of infertility are covered in this section. These include advanced age, tobacco use, alcohol intake, exposure to pollutants in the atmosphere, and particular medical conditions.

Age

Women: After the mid-30s, fertility begins to progressively drop. After the age of 37, it drastically declined since fewer and lower-quality eggs were produced.

Men: Ageing may also have an impact on sperm quality and quantity.

Alcohol Intake and Smoking: Smokers, both male and female, have an increased chance of becoming infertile. Smoking has an impact on sperm production, egg quality, and general reproductive health.

Alcohol

Drinking too much alcohol might throw off the balance of hormones and reduce fertility.

Exposure to Environmental Toxins

Long-term exposure to radiation, certain chemicals, and environmental toxins can damage reproductive organs.

Occupational Hazards: Work involving hazardous chemicals (such as welding or chemical exposure) may have an effect on fertility.

Medical Conditions

Endometriosis is an ailment whereby uterine tissue multiplies extra uterina, occasionally leading to inflammation and scarring.

Pelvic Inflammatory Disease (PID): Infertility may result from infections affecting the reproductive system. Hormonal abnormalities have an impact on ovulation in PCOS, or polycystic ovarian syndrome.

Thyroid Disorders: Thyroid issues can have an effect on infertility.

Diabetes: Improper management of diabetes may have an effect on sperm quality.

Cancer Treatment: Radiation and chemotherapy can damage reproductive cells. Recall that controlling these risk factors and seeing a specialist are crucial first steps in increasing fertility.

Identification of Infertility

An outline of the infertility diagnosis procedure is given in this section. To find the underlying reason for infertility, the diagnostic approach usually entails a physical examination, a review of medical history, and a battery of tests. Semen analysis, hormone testing, and imaging tests like hysteroscopy or ultrasound are examples of test types.

For Male

Physical Examination and Medical History: A complete examination involves an evaluation of the reproductive system, including the genitalia. The medical history aids in the identification of potential risk factors or underlying disorders. Semen analysis is an essential test to assess the health of sperm.

Samples are obtained (often by masturbating) and examined for sperm motility, count, and morphology.

Abnormalities might be a sign of problems with fertility.

Hormone Testing: Tests on the blood can quantify other male hormones, such as testosterone.

Hormonal abnormalities may have an effect on sperm production.

Genetic Testing: finds chromosomal abnormalities that might impact the development of kids or result in infertility.

Testicular Biopsy: This procedure is not often used when testing. Aids in the diagnosis of diseases that lead to infertility may also gather sperm for the purpose of in-vitro fertilisation (IVF), an assisted reproductive method.

Imaging: Ultrasound looks at the glands, sperm-carrying tubes, and scrotum brain MRIs to look for tumours of the pituitary gland that impact hormone production.

FOR FEMALE

Ovulation Assessment: Monitoring basal body temperature, menstrual cycles, and ovulation prediction devices. Hormone-level blood tests, such as progesterone testing, validate ovulation.

Hysterosalpingography (HSG): This is a contrast-enhanced X-ray that shows the uterus and fallopian tubes.
finds anomalies or obstructions.

Hysteroscopy: This minimally invasive treatment looks into the uterus using a narrow tube called a hysteroscope detects fibroids, polyps, or scar tissue.

Laparoscopy: An operation to view the organs in the pelvis recognizes tubal problems, adhesions, and endometriosis.

Hormone Testing: Determines the levels of several hormones, such as prolactin, FSH, and LH.
Detects hormone abnormalities that have an impact on fertility.

PROBLEMS WITH REPRODUCTIVE ORGANS: A CLOSER LOOK

Introduction

We explore the complex realm of reproductive organ problems in this chapter. These difficulties have an impact on men and women and influence how they become fertile. We give ourselves the ability to find possible therapies by being aware of these issues.

PolyCystic Ovarian Syndrome PCOS: Polycystic Ovary Syndrome is a prevalent hormonal condition that impacts women who are capable of bearing children. The main characteristics include several tiny cysts on the ovaries, high amounts of androgen (male hormone), and irregular menstruation periods.

Impact on Fertility: PCOS causes ovulation disturbances, which makes conception difficult. Insulin resistance and obesity are common side effects of PCOS, which further complicate fertility.

Endometriosis: Endometriosis arises from tissue growing outside the uterus that resembles the lining of the uterus. Adhesions, discomfort, and inflammation may result from it.

Effects on Fertility: Fallopian tubes, ovaries, and pelvic tissues are all impacted by endometriosis.

Tissue injury and scarring impede the movement and implantation of eggs. Options for treatment include pain management (hormonal therapy, NSAIDs). Endometrial tissue removal by laparoscopic surgery.

Varicocele: Swollen scrotal veins that impair blood flow to the testicles. It is a frequent reason for infertility in men.

Effect on Fertility: Reduced blood supply causes an elevated testicular temperature, which affects sperm production. Decreased motility and quality of sperm. Options for treatment include a varicocelectomy, a surgical procedure to enhance blood flow. Modifications to lifestyle (avoidance of heat, maintenance of a healthy weight).

Erectile Dysfunction: The inability to get or keep an erection strong enough for sexual activity is known as ED. Men of different ages are affected.

Effect on Fertility: ED patients may experience difficulty conceiving naturally as a result of sexual dysfunction.

Stress on a psychological level might make the illness worse.
Options for Treatment: Modifications to Lifestyle, Exercise, Stress Reduction and seek medical assistance.

.

FERTILITY, GENETICS, AND AGE

Introduction

We untangle the complex dance between age, genetics, and fertility in this crucial chapter. We learn more about the delicate balance that shapes our family-building journey as we delve into the scientific threads that weave our reproductive tales.

The Ovarian Symphony is for women.

Age-Related Decline: A woman's fertility starts to decline beyond the age of 35. Her ovaries, which were once full of promise, grow older with her. The orchestra that produces the eggs plays softer notes, and there are fewer ovulations on stage.

Chromosomal Abnormalities: The surviving eggs are more vulnerable to chromosomal abnormalities with the passage of time. These flaws may make it more difficult to conceive or result in an early pregnancy loss.

Health Conditions: Things like endometriosis and uterine fibroids can develop outside of the ovaries. These silent players could disturb the delicate cycle of conception.

The Paternal Baton for Men Advanced Paternal Age

Men are subject to their own time limitations. According to studies, men who are older have a higher likelihood of passing on specific genetic abnormalities to their children.

These mutations may result in birth defects or genetic diseases.

Sperm Quality: As we age, the quality of our sperm, the little messengers of life, may deteriorate. Decreased motility and damage to DNA can affect fertility.

Seeking to Discover the Right Tempo Timely Intervention: Our greatest ally is early assistance. Evaluations of fertility, counselling, and individualized advice enable us to make well-informed choices. Shared Responsibility: Keep in mind that conceiving is a joint endeavor. Mutual understanding promotes resilience, and both partners play important roles.

Fertility and Genetics the Innate Factors that Determine Our Inner Code: Our genetic make-up affects our fertility. Certain genetic diseases have a direct effect on reproductive health. Genetic Counselling: Take into account genetic counselling prior to assuming Counselling, fertility evaluations, and personalized advice help us make educated decisions. Parental responsibilities. Deciphering your own genetic code provides you with information and options. Carrier Screening: Knowledge of a carrier's status for particular situations enables couples to make informed plans. We use knowledge as a compass. In summary Let us welcome science and optimism as we navigate the landscape of ageing and genetics. Our hearts are the pen that writes our stories into our DNA. Seek knowledge, seek out relationships, and allow comprehension to guide you.

.

ALTERNATIVE THERAPIES AND LIFESTYLE CHANGES

Introduction

This chapter embraces a holistic approach to fertility, going beyond traditional treatment. By including lifestyle adjustments and complementary therapies into our story, we open up new paths for recovery and optimism.

Nutrition and Herbs

The Potential Diet for Men and Women

A nutritious diet turns our plates into canvases for fertility. The palate is composed of lean proteins, whole grains, fruits, and vegetables. Minerals, vitamins, and antioxidants support the health of our reproductive cells.

Particular Addenda: For normal cell division and foetal development, folic acid is necessary.

Zinc: Improves the quantity and quality of sperm. Increased fertility results are associated with vitamin D.

Planting the seeds of well-being

Weight management: Hormonal equilibrium is upset by excess weight. Consciously increasing or losing weight can improve fertility.

Hydration: Water satisfies the thirst of our cells as well as our own. Maintain proper hydration for best reproductive outcomes.

Harmonising the Spirit, Body, and Mind

Reduction of Stress: Yoga calms the mind and decreases cortisol levels in order to lessen stress. Stress can undermine fertility; it's our silent enemy.

Blood Flow: By increasing blood flow, yoga poses support and feeds the reproductive system. Lotus blossoms amid placid waters.

The Needles of Balance in Acupuncture

Energy Regulation: Acupuncture harmonises the body's Qi, or life force. Yin and yang are balanced when tiny needles dance along the meridians.

 Menstrual Harmony: Acupuncture helps women manage their menstrual cycles, improve ovulation, and feel less discomfort.

Sperm Quality: Sperm motility and quality are enhanced by acupuncture, which benefits men as well.

Past the Mat and Needles

Meditation: Clarity arises from silence. Soothing the spirit, meditation lowers anxiety and improves general well-being.

Herbal Treatments: Nature provides allies, from maca root to raspberry leaf tea. Speak with a herbalist for specific advice.

in conclusion
Let's welcome variety as we walk the rich roads. Holistic medicine and conventional medicine go hand in hand. May the voices of old wisdom, balance, and plenty of sustenance accompany you on your path.

FERTILITY PRESERVATION

Fertility preservation is an act of empowerment and a ray of hope for individuals walking through uncertain times. It is more than just a scientific undertaking.

Freezing of Eggs and Sperm: A Symphony of Preservation

Freezing of Eggs and Sperm: A Symphony of Preservation Oocyte Cryopreservation: Egg Freezing Imagine carefully plucking ripe fruit from a tree, each egg representing the potential for new life. Oocyte cryopreservation, commonly known as egg freezing, involves the delicate process of retrieving mature eggs from a woman's ovaries and preserving them for future use. These eggs, once harvested, are gently cradled in the cold embrace of cryopreservation, where they remain frozen in time, awaiting their destiny. Egg freezing serves as a beacon of hope in various life circumstances. For individuals undergoing cancer therapy, such as radiation or chemotherapy, which may compromise ovarian function, preserving eggs before treatment offers a chance at future fertility beyond remission. Additionally, for transgender individuals undergoing gender transition, egg freezing provides the opportunity to preserve their biological clock, allowing them to explore their gender identity without sacrificing their fertility.

Sperm Cryopreservation: Sperm Freezing

In a similar vein, sperm cryopreservation, or sperm freezing, halts the journey of these tiny life travelers midway, ensuring their preservation for future use. Sperm, often likened to the "seed of life," undergo cryopreservation where they are safeguarded from the threat of frostbite by cryoprotectants. These resilient fighters rest in a state of suspended animation within liquid nitrogen, awaiting the call to action. Sperm freezing proves invaluable in various life scenarios. Men undergoing medical operations, such as cancer surgery or therapies, can safeguard their fertility by preserving sperm beforehand. Similarly, individuals making life decisions, whether embarking on daring adventures or choosing to spend time alone, can take comfort in knowing that their fertility remains preserved through sperm freezing. In essence, both oocyte cryopreservation and sperm cryopreservation

offer individuals the opportunity to safeguard their fertility in the face
of life's uncertainties, providing a beacon of hope for the future.

The Purpose of Maintaining Fertility

Preserving fertility serves as a beacon of hope, offering individuals the
opportunity to shape their genetic legacy, find solace in uncertainty, and
make informed decisions about their reproductive health.

Biological Legacy: Preserving fertility provides a blank canvas for our
genetic heritage to paint its masterpiece on. Each preserved egg or
sperm represents the potential for new life, allowing individuals to pass
on their genetic legacy to future generations. In a world where our
stories matter, preserving fertility ensures that our genetic voice
continues to resonate long after we're gone.

Calm in the Face of Uncertainty: During times of illness or medical
procedures, maintaining fertility serves as a link to the future and a
source of calm. Knowing that fertility is preserved offers reassurance
and comfort, providing individuals with a sense of continuity amidst
life's uncertainties. It allows them to envision a future where they can
still pursue their dreams of parenthood, even in the face of adversity.

Making Informed Decisions: Information serves as our guide on the
journey of reproductive health. By assuming responsibility for
maintaining fertility, individuals empower themselves to make informed
decisions about their future. Whether considering egg freezing or sperm
cryopreservation, seeking advice from reproductive professionals
ensures that choices are tailored to each individual's unique
circumstances and aspirations.

ETHICAL ASPECTS OF REPRODUCTIVE MEDICINE

This section introduces the chapter by highlighting the ethical complexities inherent in reproductive medicine. It emphasizes the importance of making decisions that uphold both scientific principles and human values. Readers are encouraged to explore these ethical dilemmas as they navigate the subsequent discussions.

The Mutual Understanding

Pact Informed Consent: Beyond a simple signature, informed consent involves a comprehensive discussion between healthcare providers and patients. It ensures that patients fully understand the risks, benefits, and available options for their treatment, empowering them to make informed decisions.

Receiving Progress in Moral Situations: This emphasizes the importance of transparency in communication between healthcare providers and patients. It stresses the need for patients to have the capacity to understand their options, enabling them to participate in decision-making processes that respect their autonomy.

Autonomy with Dignity: The Right to Self-Determination This section underscores the fundamental principle of patient autonomy, which extends beyond legal definitions. It emphasizes the importance of respecting patients' cultural backgrounds, values, and beliefs while also finding a balance between providing information and honoring their autonomy.

Fairness Concerns: The focus is on the ethical considerations surrounding resource allocation in fertility treatments. It advocates for an equitable distribution of resources to ensure that everyone has access to reproductive care, regardless of financial status. However, it also acknowledges the ethical dilemmas that arise when demand exceeds supply.

The Emotional Terrain: This section delves into the emotional impact of fertility treatments and the importance of managing expectations. It acknowledges the range of emotions evoked by these treatments and emphasizes the need to balance hope with reality. Providing robust support systems is highlighted as crucial for individuals navigating these emotional challenges. The conclusion emphasizes the importance of respecting individual choices while navigating the ethical complexities of reproductive medicine. It encourages readers to approach these dilemmas with kindness, openness, and respect, recognizing the essence of humanity at the intersection of science and ethics.

MOVING FORWARD

The emotional terrain of infertility challenges is called to embrace in Chapter Eight, as we find ourselves at the intersection of hope and perseverance. Here, we acknowledge the emotional rollercoaster that goes along with this journey and throw light on the shadows. Let's proceed with kindness, discernment, and open hearts.

Acknowledging and Comprehending the Emotional Wave

The Unseen Waves: Infertility is an emotional journey as much as a physical illness. Identify the waves, the peaks, and the valleys of optimism and sorrow. Honest Communication Hold hands, partners. Tell the truth about what you know. Talk about your dreams, doubts, and anxieties. The trip on the emotional rollercoaster is in pairs.

Seeking professional advice: Professional counsellors provide a compass for navigating emotional storms. They support us in overcoming uncertainty, worry, and sadness.

Support Groups: Get together with other travelers. Our common weakness gives us strength.

Self-Care: Soul-Nourishing

Methods of Relaxation: Take deep breaths, Think and Calm the nervous system down. Nature walks, soothing music, and warm baths are not indulgences; they are necessities.

Creative pastimes: painting, dancing, writing, or gardening. Hobbies whisper to the soul. Creativity offers us comfort.

The Self-Love Cup: Put the rest first. Heart medication takes the form of sleep. Feed your body and soul with nutrition. One of the languages of love is nourishment.
Limits: Take care of your vitality. When necessary, say no.

How Infertility Affects Relationships

Communication: Pay attention, partners. Talk. Feel the weight of loss and yearning together.

Patience: Infertility puts relationships to the test. Show each other compassion when grieving.

Seeking Professional Assistance: Couples therapy offers strategies for negotiating emotional minefields. In summary let's honor our hearts as we proceed. May we discover resilience in the face of uncertainty, grace in connection, and strength in vulnerability. Never forget that you are not   alone   in   every   step   you   take

.

ASSISTED REPRODUCTIVE TECHNOLOGIES (ART) AND MEDICAL INTERVENTIONS

As we venture into the realm of medical interventions, Chapter Nine acts as a compass, directing us through the confusing world of reproductive treatments. Here, hope and science combine to provide routes to parenting. Allow us to simplify the intricacies so that you are capable of making wise decisions.

Diagnostic Assessments

Fertility Assessment: Diagnostic tests are the first step in the process. Semen analysis, blood tests, and ultrasounds show the picture of your fertility. A radiologic technique called hysterosalpingography (HSG) is used to examine the uterus and fallopian tubes.

Genetic testing: deciphering genetic enigmas that might influence fertility.

Medications: Managing Hormones

Drugs for Fertility: The name Clomid (Clomiphene Citrate) encourages the release of eggs from the ovaries by stimulating ovulation. Although not recognized as fertility medications, Femara (letrozole) and Arimidex (anastrozole) both coincide with ovulation. Gonadotropins are hormones that stimulate the creation of eggs.

Surgical Procedures: Accuracy and Hope

The art of the Surgeon: Hysteroscopy and laparoscopy are minimally invasive techniques used to detect and treat uterine abnormalities, fibroids, and endometriosis

.

Varicocelectomy: for males whose swollen veins impair the quality of their sperm. Repairing damaged or obstructed fallopian tubes is known as tubal surgery.

Technologies for Assisted Reproduction (ART)

Intrauterine Insemination (IUI): A closer meeting of the sperm and the eggs. IVF (in vitro fertilization) is the big orchestra. After retrieving the eggs, sperm is added, the embryos are cultivated in a lab, and finally the uterine stage is reached. When sperm require a special pass to enter the egg, this is known as intracytoplasmic sperm injection or ICSI. Freezing embryos for later use is known as embryo cryopreservation.

The distinctions between IVF and IUI

Intrauterine insemination or IUI:

Procedure: The uterus is immediately injected with sperm. Increases the sperm's probability of reaching the eggs by reducing the distance they must travel.

Process: To separate sperm from seminal fluid, a semen sample is washed. The uterus receives a direct injection of the complete sperm sample.

Timing: performed the day following a spike in ovulation it usually takes ten to fifteen minutes.

Indications: used to treat cervical problems, minor male factor infertility, and infertility without apparent cause. Occasionally in conjunction with ovulation induction.

Success rate: varies, although it's usually not as high as with IVF.

In vitro fertilization or IVF:

Process: The ovaries create many follicles (containing eggs) in response to high-dose hormone stimulation. Retrieving eggs requires outpatient surgery. In a lab, donor or partner sperm is mixed with eggs. The resultant embryos are either kept for later use or inserted into the uterus.

Indications: used to treat a variety of infertility problems, such as endometriosis, severe male factor infertility, tubal obstruction, and infertility that cannot be explained.

Success rate: It is typically greater than that of IUI. A number of variables, including age, ovarian reserve, and general health, affect success. In conclusion IUI injects sperm straight into the uterus, whereas IVF requires a more involved process. Infertility patients might find hope with both therapies, which are based on personal circumstances and   medical   guidance.

MODIFICATIONS TO LIFESTYLE AND ALTERNATIVE THERAPIES

This chapter explores medicinal methods, alternative therapies, and lifestyle modifications that can support people in their efforts to become fertile. Our objective is to provide readers with a wide range of alternatives so they may make well-informed decisions according to their own circumstances.

Boosting Fertility

An Equitable Diet: Eating a well-balanced diet is essential for maximizing fertility in both men and women. Key nutritional factors are as follows: -

Vegetables and fruits: These vibrant powerhouses supply vital minerals, vitamins, and antioxidants. A variety of fruit should be your goal to meet all nutritional needs.

Whole Grains: Use whole grains such as oats, brown rice, and quinoa. They regulate blood sugar and improve general well-being.

Lean Protein: Choose tofu, fish, chicken, and lentils as your lean protein sources. Protein aids in the formation of sperm and eggs. Consume foods high in healthy fats, such as almonds, avocados, and olive oil. These lipids are necessary for the synthesis of hormones.

Particular Additives: Fertility can be improved by taking certain vitamins. Never forget to get medical advice before beginning any new routine.

Folic Acid: An essential nutrient for foetal growth, folic acid lowers the chance of neural tube abnormalities. It's quite important for ladies who intend to get pregnant.

Zinc: This mineral helps to maintain the quality and quantity of sperm. Nuts, whole grains, and oysters are among the foods high in zinc.

Vitamin D: Better reproductive outcomes are linked to adequate amounts of vitamin D. You can satisfy your requirements with fortified meals and sun exposure.

Complementary approaches in alternative therapies

Yoga: Linking Mind and Body

Stress Reduction: Yoga lowers stress hormones, which is good for your health in general. Stress has a big impact on fertility, so consider practicing gentle yoga poses.
Enhanced Blood Flow: Certain asanas improve blood flow to the reproductive system. Pose variations that might be helpful include Legs Up-the-Wall (Viparita Karani) and Butterfly (Baddha Konasana).

Harmonizing Energies

Menstrual cycle control: Acupuncture's effect on hormone balance may help regulate erratic cycles. Women with polycystic ovarian syndrome (PCOS) benefit most from it.
Improving Sperm Quality: Research indicates that acupuncture could help with sperm motility and general health.

Meditation: Mindfulness techniques ease tension and encourage calmness. Think about including meditation in your everyday schedule.

Hypnosis: For some people, hypnosis is an effective way to deal with anxiety associated with fertility treatments.

Herbal Remedies: For secure and scientifically supported herbal remedies, speak with a herbalist. Certain herbs, such as maca root and chasteberry (Vitex), have been linked to improved fertility. Recall that every person's journey is distinct. Investigate these complementary therapies in addition to traditional ones, and always get expert advice. You may handle infertility with empathy and optimism if you combine holistic practices with well-informed decisions. Making the decision to see a fertility expert is a crucial first step. The following techniques will assist you in making a connection with an informed and sympathetic healthcare provider

Look up fertility clinics online: Fertility clinics vary from one another to investigate respectable clinics in your neighborhood first. Seek out reproductive medicine specialists with a solid track record of care. Go to the Society for Assisted Reproductive Technology's (SART) website. They offer data on the success rates of IVF treatments at different facilities.

Verify Credentials: Verify the fertility specialist's board certification in infertility and reproductive endocrinology. Seek out medical professionals who belong to associations such as the American Society for Reproductive Medicine (ASRM).

Examine comments and suggestions: Consult your family, friends, and online groups for recommendations. It might be beneficial to learn about the experiences of others. Look into internet forums where patients discuss and exchange opinions about particular fertility physicians or facilities.

Speak with your insurance company: To find out if fertility treatments are covered by your health insurance, get in touch with them. They are able to offer an inventory of in-network experts. Verify if treatments, diagnostic procedures, and consultations are covered.

Visit centers for fertility: Make appointments to speak with a few reproductive clinics. Inquire about their methods, success rates, and available treatments during these visits. Talk about your particular circumstances and any worries you may have. Think about accessibility and location. Pick a clinic that is easily accessible to you and in a convenient location. Throughout therapy, it may be necessary to make frequent visits.

Inquire about available treatment options: Find out what kinds of therapies are available. Does the clinic provide other therapies like egg freezing, IUI, and surrogacy in addition to IVF? If you're interested, talk about holistic methods and alternative remedies.
Embrace your gut feelings: Throughout your conversations with the fertility professional, be mindful of your feelings. Comfort and trust are important on this delicate trip.

FERTILITY PRESERVATION THROUGH FREEZING EGGS AND SPERM

This chapter covers the important subject of freezing eggs and sperm to preserve fertility. Knowing about these processes can enable you to make educated decisions regarding your reproductive health, regardless of whether you're starting treatment for cancer, dealing with a medical issue, or changing your gender.

The Method

Gathering Eggs: The first step in egg freezing is taking the eggs out of the ovaries of women. It is usual practice to do this sensitive treatment under anesthesia.

Cryopreservation: Using cutting-edge cryoprotectants, the collected eggs are then carefully frozen. You may keep these frozen eggs for many years.

Eventually Use: The frozen eggs can be fertilized with sperm when the moment is appropriate, either because of medical procedures or individual circumstances, to produce embryos for assisted reproductive methods such as in vitro fertilization (IVF).

Cancer Therapy: Radiation and chemotherapy can impair ovarian function. There is hope for future fertility when eggs are preserved prior to therapy.

Gender Transition: Before beginning hormone therapy, transgender people can preserve their biological potential by freezing their eggs.

Semen Collection: Masturbating is how guys give a sample of their semen. Next, the quality of the sperm in the sample is assessed. Sperm cryopreservation involves the use of specific procedures, similar to egg freezing. After freezing, it doesn't lose its viability.

Eventually Use: Sperm that has been thawed can be used for IVF or intrauterine insemination (IUI). Situations in which sperm freeze:

Medical Conditions: Sperm freezing is a way for men undergoing cancer treatments or surgery to protect their fertility.

Occupational Risks: People in the military, firefighters, and other high-risk occupations may decide to freeze their sperm as a precaution.

Making Empowering Decisions

Biological Parenthood: When the timing is perfect, freezing eggs and sperm may allow for the potential of biological offspring.

Peace of Mind: During difficult medical treatments, it is emotionally comforting to know that fertility is protected.

Control Over Reproductive Health: People may reclaim control over their reproductive fate by being proactive.

Speak with a medical professional: Speak candidly with a fertility professional before pursuing egg or sperm freezing. Recognize the advantages, disadvantages, and probable consequences. Your selections will be based on your particular situation. Recall that fertility preservation is about more than just science; it's also about optimism, fortitude, and the promise of the future.

Let's clear up some myths regarding freezing sperm and eggs

Myth: It Takes a Complex Process to Freeze Eggs
Facts: Freezing eggs is a multi-step, reasonably simple process.

Hormonal drugs stimulate the ovaries, increasing the quantity of eggs that are accessible.

Monitoring: evaluating the size and maturity of the eggs.
Retrieval of Eggs: A minimally intrusive method for gathering mature eggs.
Cryopreservation: Vitrification is used to freeze eggs.

Storage: Until they are required for in vitro fertilization (IVF), eggs are stored at low temperatures.
Myth: It's Not Safe to Freeze Eggs
Facts: Although egg freezing is usually safe, ovarian stimulation drugs may cause uncomfortable side effects, including bloating. Medical professionals closely monitor and very rarely experience severe

consequences (e.g., ovarian hyperstimulation syndrome).

Myth: Egg Freezing Affects Natural Fertility

Facts: Freezing eggs doesn't lower your natural egg production. People naturally lose eggs over time; egg freezing protects the ones that are already there. It doesn't hasten the depletion of viable eggs.

Myth: There Are No Harmful Effects from Storing Sperm indefinitely

Facts: Although sperm may be kept in storage for a long time, it's important to follow the right procedures. One risk is possible damage during thawing or extended storage. Regular checkups ensure high-quality sperm. Recall that fertility preservation gives people the power to decide for themselves what is best for their reproductive health. See a healthcare professional for advice on any particular issues or queries you may have.

Treatments for Fertility with Ethical Considerations

Making informed decisions

We acknowledge that assisted reproductive technologies (ART) carry significant ethical issues when you begin the complex process of undergoing fertility treatments. We want to empower your choices, provide you with new perspectives, and promote mutual understanding. Let's examine the salient points:

Openness and voluntary knowledge

Transparency: This is our compass while talking about fertility treatments. Patients have a right to accurate information on prices, success rates, hazards, and treatments. The crucial procedure of "informed consent" guarantees that people are completely aware of the effects of the decisions they make. Practitioners have candid conversations about the advantages and possible disadvantages. It is important to keep in mind that informed consent serves as a link between patient empowerment and medical knowledge.

Honoring Individuality and Initiative

Autonomy: Choosing a fertility treatment offers a plethora of personal options. We respect your autonomy, or your choice to accept or reject specific interventions.

Avoiding Paternalism: Medical professionals avoid having a paternalistic mindset. Rather, you are actively involved in the design of your therapy. Making decisions together increases trust and gives you power. Your opinions count. It matters what you choose.

Emotional Support and Psychological Effects

The Price of Infertility: Individuals and couples are both impacted by the emotional rollercoaster. We comprehend your disappointment, hope, and fear.

Psychological Support: During this phase, make connections with support groups and look for therapy services. You are not alone. Recall that the feeling is OK. When in doubt, seek comfort.

Handling Anticipations Handling Difficulties: Emotional pain can result from unrealistic expectations. Adopt pragmatic optimism. Honor advancement, even if it's not the end goal. We manage the fine line between hope and resilience together. In conclusion, as you peruse these pages, keep in mind that morality plays a role in every choice you make. We are here to support you on this special journey of yours. Together, let's walk this route with empathy, comprehension, and unflinching support.

ACCEPTING SENSITIVITY AND RESILIENCY

We encourage you to embrace vulnerability in this book and the bravery to be honest despite life's obstacles. Resilience is also significant. It's not about avoiding suffering, but rather about getting stronger and learning from each setback.

Pathways to Becoming a Parent

Adoption: Beyond Biology, Love Is Selecting Adoption. Adoption is a lovely family-building strategy. It is centered on love and goes beyond biology.

Adoptive Parents: These amazing people provide needy children with secure, loving environments. Parenting is not only about blood relations.

Fostering Biological ties through Surrogacy

When conception is impossible: It is possible for intended parents to become parents through surrogacy. To bridge the gap between hope and reality, a surrogate bears the pregnancy selflessly.

Creating Connections via Similar Experiences

Different Forms: Families can take on a variety of forms, including mixed families and stepfamilies. Love has no bounds.

Shared Experiences: Through perseverance, humor, and shared moments, mixed families forge relationships.

Realization Occurs

Partnerships: Valued Connections, families, friends, and partners. Developing relationships is just as important as being a parent. It values the connections that keep you going.

Self-Growth: Investing in Personal Development Passions and Purpose. Finding fulfillment comes from more than just parenthood. Invest in your interests, take up new hobbies, and discover a purpose outside of the nursery.

Engaging the Community: Having an Impact beyond your circle. Get involved in your community, have a good impact, and leave a legacy that extends beyond your own family.

Moving Ahead: The road to life is complex. Parenthood is a significant chapter in life, but it's not the only one. Accept understanding, resiliency, and optimism. The future holds a plethora of opportunities. Recall that experiences, relationships, and personal development comprise the rich fabric of life, in addition to biology, and are what lead to fulfillment.

ABOUT THE AUTHOR

Dr. Whitney David PhD, is a psychologist and She has specialized in infertility since 2004 and has served on the regional board of RESOLVE, the National Infertility Organization.

Dr. Whitney David is a published author, featured speaker, and workshop facilitator. Drawing from the lessons of her own journey through infertility and those of the women and men she has worked with.

Dr. Whitney David brings the teaching and practice of mindfulness to the challenge of fertility. Her book, "Fertile Path: navigating infertility with understanding and hope, Guiding the Journey with Mindfulness and Compassion," provides practical strategies, exercises, and meditations to help individuals develop resilience during their fertility journey.

Dr. Whitney David emphasizes the mind-body connection in fertility and recognizes that emotional well-being, stress reduction, and self-nurturance are essential components of the fertility process. She is a graduate of Yale University and the University of Nevada, Reno.

Dr. Whitney David's work bridges the gap between psychology, mindfulness, and fertility. She advocates for a holistic approach to fertility, her book provides practical strategies, exercises, and meditations to help individuals develop resilience during their fertility.

www.ingramcontent.com/pod-product-compliance
Lightning Source LLC
Chambersburg PA
CBHW070752260726
48660CB00007B/3085